CHEMICAL PEELS FOR BEGINNERS

Transform Skin With Safe & Effective Techniques For Acne, Wrinkles, And Hyperpigmentation

DR SAWYER DIEGO

DISCLAMER

Nothing in this book should be interpreted as medical advice; it is meant exclusively for educational reasons. Regarding their specific health issues and treatment options, readers are urged to speak with licensed healthcare professionals. The publisher and author disclaim all liability for any errors or omissions in the material provided, as well as for any negative effects that may arise from using or abusing the information. Although every attempt has been taken to guarantee that the material in this book is correct as of the date of publishing, new research may have superseded some of the content because medical knowledge is always changing. It is recommended that readers confirm the most recent medical recommendations and guidelines. The reader of this book undertakes to release the author and publisher from any claims or liabilities resulting from the use of this information, and understands and accepts the inherent risks connected with healthcare decisions.

TABLE OF CONTENTS

ABOUT THE BOOK

The book "Chemical Peels for Beginners" is an invaluable resource for anyone wishing to explore the world of chemical peels for skincare enhancement. It covers all aspects of chemical peels in detail, starting with an extensive introduction that explains the basic principles underlying these treatments.

 Knowing the fundamentals of chemical peels is important because it lays the foundation for realizing their transformative potential on the skin. Stressing the significance of skin preparation highlights how appropriate pre-peel care can maximize results and minimize risks, guaranteeing a safe and efficient procedure.

Exploring the various kinds of chemical peels, the book covers superficial, medium, and deep peels and clarifies the variations in ingredients like AHAs, BHAs, TCAs, and phenol. This comprehensive study helps readers choose the best peel depending on their skin type and sensitivity; it also assures them of the risks and side effects, giving them the knowledge they need to approach peels with caution and confidence.

To ensure that people approach their skincare journey with informed optimism, the book devotes an entire chapter to guiding readers through consultation processes, pre-peel skincare regimens, and lifestyle adjustments that may influence outcomes. Setting realistic goals and managing expectations further enrich this preparatory phase.

Whether the procedure is done professionally or at home using DIY kits, the reader's understanding of the subtleties of the procedure is enhanced by practical advice on comfort measures, pain management strategies, and monitoring skin reactions. Detailed step-by-step breakdowns and insights into what to expect during the peel procedure itself provide a reassuring roadmap.

The book provides thorough advice on immediate skincare routines, long-term considerations, and measures like sun protection.

Post-peel care and recovery are equally important, and this holistic approach not only helps healing but also encourages sustained skin health between peel sessions.

A deeper understanding of the safety and benefits of chemical peels is fostered by addressing common concerns and dispelling myths about them. Advice on how to manage post-peel sensations, deal with unexpected reactions, and get ready for follow-up sessions guarantees that readers feel empowered and informed throughout their skincare journey.

Budget considerations and safety precautions for at-home peels highlight the book's commitment to ensuring safe and accessible skincare practices. Whether considering professional treatments or do-it-yourself options, readers benefit from a nuanced exploration of the pros and cons associated with each approach.

Comprehensive FAQs anticipate and address frequently asked questions, from peel strength selection to considerations during pregnancy, enhancing the book's value as a reliable resource for skincare education. Advanced tips for optimizing peel results, integrating complementary skincare treatments, and tailoring peels to specific skin concerns elevate the book's utility for both novice and seasoned users alike.

Looking ahead, the exploration of future trends in peel formulations, emerging technologies and sustainable practices reflects the book's commitment to staying abreast of industry advancements. Educational resources and global perspectives on skincare trends further empower readers to make informed decisions about their skincare regimens, fostering a proactive approach to personal skin health and rejuvenation.

CHAPTER ONE
CHEMICAL PEELS OVERVIEW
KNOWING THE FUNDAMENTALS OF CHEMICAL PEELS

Chemical peels are a class of dermatological treatments that target the outermost layer (epidermis) and are best suited for mild skin imperfections. Superficial peels target the outermost layer (epidermis) and are ideal for more moderate skin imperfections. Medium and deep peels penetrate deeper layers, treating more severe skin issues like wrinkles and scars. The chemical solution is applied to the skin and causes controlled exfoliation, effectively removing outer layers of damaged or dead skin cells, revealing smoother and rejuvenated skin underneath.

Understanding the basics includes knowing what skin conditions chemical peels can treat, how they work, and their potential benefits. The process usually entails cleansing the skin, applying the chemical solution for a set amount of time, and then neutralizing it to stop the exfoliation process. Post-treatment care involves moisturizing and protecting the skin from sun exposure to maximize healing and results.

Before having a chemical peel, it's imperative to speak with a dermatologist to determine the most suitable type based on your skin type, concerns, and desired outcomes.

THE SIGNIFICANCE OF SKIN CARE

Skincare products containing retinoid or alpha hydroxyl acids (AHAs) may also be suggested by dermatologists to prime the skin in the weeks before the chemical peel, as these products help to accelerate cell turnover and enhance the results of the peel. Proper skin preparation involves cleansing the skin thoroughly to remove dirt, oils, and makeup. This ensures that the chemical solution can penetrate evenly and deeply into the skin layers, promoting a more uniform exfoliation process.

Prioritizing skin preparation allows people to maximize the results of chemical peels, attain smoother skin texture, and reduce the risk of negative reactions. Avoiding excessive sun exposure and using sunscreen daily are also important aspects of skin preparation, as sun-damaged skin is more sensitive and prone to complications during and after a chemical peel. Adequate hydration is also crucial, as hydrated skin tends to heal faster and experience fewer side effects post-peel.

SAFETY POINTS TO REMEMBER

Even though chemical peels are generally safe when done by qualified professionals, there are some important safety things to keep in mind. First and foremost, it's important to choose the right type and strength of peel for your skin type and concerns. Superficial peels usually have less downtime and are safer, so they're good for beginners and people with sensitive skin. On the other hand, medium and deep peels require more recovery time and may lead to higher risks of complications like infection and changes in pigmentation, so a dermatologist should evaluate them carefully.

It is common to feel tingling or burning during the procedure as the chemical solution interacts with the skin; however, excessive pain, blistering, or severe redness should be reported right away to the healthcare provider. After treatment, the treated area should be gently cleaned, moisturized, and kept clean to prevent infection and scarring. Following these safety instructions guarantees a more comfortable recovery and lowers the risk of negative reactions, which increases patient satisfaction with the peel's outcomes.

AN OVERVIEW OF THE VARIOUS PEEL TYPES

Different chemical peels have different strengths and depths that allow for flexibility in treating different skin concerns. Superficial peels, like glycolic acid or salicylic acid, are mild, mostly targeting fine lines, dullness, and acne; they require little recovery time and are appropriate for most skin types. Medium peels, like TCA, are deeper and target moderate wrinkles, sun damage, and pigment irregularities; they may cause swelling and require recovery time ranging from a few days to a week.

Deciding which type of peel to get depends on your desired results, skin type, and tolerance for downtime. Consulting with a dermatologist ensures that you select the safest and most effective peel tailored to your specific needs. Deep peels, like phenol peels, provide the most dramatic results by reaching the deeper layers of the skin. They are effective for treating severe wrinkles, scars, and precancerous growths but involve significant downtime and are generally reserved for specific skin concerns under strict medical supervision.

ADVANTAGES AND ANTICIPATIONS

Expectations should be reasonable, with noticeable improvements usually evident after a series of peels spaced several weeks apart. Results vary depending on the type of peel, skin condition, and individual response, necessitating adherence to post-peel care instructions for optimal healing and maintenance. The benefits of chemical peels stretch beyond aesthetic improvements to include enhanced skin texture, reduction in fine lines, improved skin tone, and minimized acne scars.

A positive experience and satisfactory results from chemical peel treatments are ensured when patients understand these benefits and manage their expectations. In the short term, patients can expect temporary redness, flaking, and mild irritation immediately after the peel, which usually subsides within a few days. Sun protection is crucial during the healing phase to prevent hyperpigmentation and maintain results. In the long term, ongoing skin rejuvenation and a more youthful appearance with continued skincare maintenance.

CHAPTER TWO

CHEMICAL PEELS: WHAT ARE THEY?

DEFINITION AND OBJECTIVE

By applying a chemical solution to the skin, chemical peels are cosmetic treatments that aim to improve the texture and appearance of the skin. The main goal of chemical peels is to exfoliate the skin's outer layers, encouraging the shedding of dead skin cells and stimulating cellular turnover.

This process helps to reveal smoother, more youthful-looking skin beneath the surface and can address a variety of skin concerns like sun damage, uneven pigmentation, fine lines, and acne scars. Chemical peels also encourage the production of collagen by removing damaged skin layers, which can eventually result in firmer, more youthful-looking skin.

The depth of a chemical peel determines its effects and recovery time; deeper peels require longer healing periods but offer more dramatic results.

Chemical peels range in strength from superficial to deep, depending on the specific skin issues being targeted. Superficial peels usually use milder acids like alpha hydroxy acids (AHAs) or beta hydroxy acids (BHAs), while deeper peels may involve stronger acids like trichloroacetic acid (TCA) or phenol.

Knowing why a chemical peel is beneficial means realizing that it can revitalize the skin's appearance by eliminating damaged layers and encouraging healthier skin growth. Depending on the type and depth of the peel, people can achieve better tone, smoother texture, and fewer signs of sun damage or aging. Speaking with a dermatologist or skincare specialist is essential to figuring out which type of chemical peel is best for their specific skin concerns and objectives.

HOW CHEMICAL SKIN PEELS OPERATE

Depending on the type and strength of the peel, the specific acids used in the solution penetrate the skin to varying depths; superficial peels target the epidermis, while deeper peels can reach into the dermis, the deeper layer of skin. The application of a chemical solution to the skin causes controlled damage to the outer layers, which triggers the skin's natural healing response, stimulating the production of new skin cells and collagen.

Following the chemical solution application, there may be noticeable peeling or flaking of the skin as the damaged layers shed over several days to a week. This shedding process reveals smoother, more youthful-looking skin underneath, with fewer imperfections and an improved texture. Over time, the chemical peels' exfoliating effects can also help to unclog pores, lessen the appearance of fine lines and wrinkles, and lessen the appearance of acne breakouts.

The effectiveness of chemical peels can vary depending on factors like the type of acid used, the concentration of the solution, and individual skin characteristics. It is imperative to adhere to post-peel care instructions provided by a skincare professional to maximize results and minimize potential side effects like redness or sensitivity. Regular use of sunscreen and moisturization is typically recommended post-peel to protect the newly exposed skin and maintain its improved appearance.

SKIN CONDITIONS THEY TREAT

Superficial peels like glycolic or salicylic acid are good for mild acne, dull complexion, and uneven skin tone. Chemical peels are adaptable treatments that can address a variety of common skin concerns and conditions. They are especially effective for improving skin texture, reducing acne scars, and diminishing hyperpigmentation caused by sun damage or hormonal changes.

Those with sun-damaged skin, melasma (patchy brown discoloration), or moderate to severe acne scarring may benefit from deeper chemical peels for more noticeable results. Deeper peels, like those using TCA or phenol, can effectively smooth deeper wrinkles, reduce age spots, and improve overall skin texture and tone. These peels penetrate more deeply into the skin layers, promoting significant collagen remodeling and enhancing skin elasticity over time.

Understanding the types of conditions that chemical peels can treat helps people make educated decisions about improving their skin's health and appearance through professional skincare treatments. Selecting the right type of chemical peel depends on the specific skin concerns and the desired outcome. Consulting with a qualified dermatologist or skincare professional is crucial to determine the most appropriate treatment plan tailored to individual needs and skin type.

SKIN TYPES THAT WORK WELL WITH CHEMICAL PEELS

Chemical peels can be helpful for a variety of skin types, but the type of peel that is best for you will depend on your unique skin type and its characteristics. Superficial peels, on the other hand, are safe for most skin types, even sensitive skin, and can improve skin texture and provide gentle exfoliation without causing significant irritation or downtime.

Salicylic acid peels can help unclog pores and minimize acne breakouts in people with oily or acne-prone skin. Superficial peels are also appropriate for people with uneven skin tone, mild sun damage, or fine lines. They are frequently prescribed as maintenance treatments to keep the skin looking young and refreshed.

Consultation with a skincare professional is essential to assess skin type and determine the safest and most effective peel option for achieving desired skin improvements. Deeper chemical peels, like those using TCA or phenol, are more suitable for people with fair to medium skin tones and specific skin concerns like deep wrinkles, significant sun damage, or acne scarring. These peels penetrate deeper into the skin layers and may require longer recovery times compared to superficial peels.

FACTORS AFFECTING THE EFFECTIVENESS OF PEEL

The type, concentration, and depth of penetration into the skin layers are some of the factors that determine how effective chemical peels are. Superficial peels, on the other hand, usually have milder effects and may require multiple treatments to gradually achieve desired results. They are appropriate for people who want mild exfoliation and improvement in skin tone and texture without a significant amount of downtime.

The effectiveness of a chemical peel also depends on the type of skin, sensitivity, and presence of specific skin concerns such as acne scars or hyperpigmentation. Consulting with a qualified skincare professional ensures that the chosen peel matches individual needs and goals for skin improvement. Deeper chemical peels, on the other hand, offer more dramatic results but involve greater risks and longer recovery periods.

Proper skincare before and after treatment helps to optimize results, minimize potential side effects, and support skin healing and regeneration. Sunscreen use, moisturization, and avoiding excessive sun exposure are essential aspects of maintaining skin health and preserving the benefits of chemical peel treatments over time. Pre-peel preparation and post-peel care routines significantly impact the overall effectiveness and safety of chemical peels.

CHAPTER THREE

CHEMICAL PEEL TYPES

AN EXPLANATION OF SUPERFICIAL, MEDIUM, AND DEEP PEELS

Chemical peels are available in different strengths and depths, each designed to target specific skin concerns. The mildest types of chemical peels are called superficial peels, and they mainly target the epidermis, using gentle acids like lactic acid or glycolic acid, which are alpha hydroxyl acids (AHAs). These peels are ideal for beginners and those seeking a quick skin refresh as they help improve skin texture, reduce fine lines, and enhance brightness with little downtime.

A combination of acids, such as beta hydroxyl acids and trichloroacetic acid (TCA) at higher concentrations, is often used in medium peels, which reach the middle layer (dermis) of the skin and can address more prominent wrinkles, pigmentation problems, and mild to moderate skin imperfections.

Recovery from medium peels is longer than that of superficial peels, and some redness and peeling may occur for a few days after the procedure.

Deep peels are the strongest and target the deepest layers of the skin. They are usually performed under sedation due to discomfort, and they require careful planning. Deep peels are the most intense and penetrate the deepest layers of the skin; often involving phenol, a strong acid that effectively treats severe sun damage, deep wrinkles, and significant skin discoloration. Recovery from deep peels can take weeks, during which the skin experiences significant peeling and redness before revealing smoother, rejuvenated skin.

VARIATIONS IN THE INGREDIENTS (TCA, PHENOL, BHAS, AND AHAS)

Comprehending the components of chemical peels aids in choosing the appropriate course of action for individual skin concerns. Alpha hydroxyl acids (AHAs), such as lactic acid and glycolic acid, are frequently found in superficial peels; they provide mild exfoliation and improve skin brightness and texture, making them appropriate for treating mild discoloration and fine lines.

When combined with alpha hydroxyl acids (AHAs) for medium-depth peels, beta hydroxyl acids (BHAs)—like salicylic acid—go deeper into the pores and are therefore useful in treating oily skin, blackheads, and acne. This provides a more thorough approach to treating uneven texture and acne-prone skin.

Trichloroacetic acid (TCA) is a versatile ingredient that is used in medium-depth peels to address mild skin flaws such as sun damage, uneven pigmentation, and fine wrinkles. Compared to AHAs and BHAs, TCA offers a more powerful exfoliation that promotes the creation of collagen and skin renewal.

The most potent ingredient in deep chemical peels, phenol penetrates the skin deeply to treat deep wrinkles, scars, and severe sun damage. Because of their potency and potential side effects, which can include skin lightening and longer recovery times, phenol peels must be applied and monitored carefully.

SELECTING THE APPROPRIATE PEEL FOR YOUR SKIN ISSUES

A superficial peel with AHAs or a mild combination of AHAs and BHAs can enhance skin texture and luminosity and offer gentle exfoliation for beginners and people with modest skin concerns. The choice of chemical peel relies on your unique skin concerns and desired results.

A medium-depth peel using TCA or a combination of AHAs and BHAs may be appropriate for you if you have moderate skin imperfections such as mild wrinkles, uneven skin tone, or acne scars.

These peels offer deeper penetration to address more significant concerns while promoting collagen production and skin renewal.

A deep peel with phenol might be considered for people with severe sun damage, deep wrinkles, or pigmentation problems. Deep peels are intense and come with risks, so dermatologists usually advise against them unless they are thoroughly evaluated.

POSSIBLE DANGERS AND ADVERSE REACTIONS

Superficial peels usually have low risks, like transient redness or mild irritation, which usually go away in a few days. Chemical peels, on the other hand, can cause significant improvements in the quality of your skin, but they also come with risks and side effects.

More noticeable side effects from medium-depth peels include redness, swelling, and increased photosensitivity. In rare instances, medium-depth peels can result in infection or hyperpigmentation if proper post-treatment care is not received.

It is important to carefully follow post-peel care instructions to minimize risks and ensure optimal healing.

Deep peels are the most likely to cause side effects, including prolonged redness, swelling, and peeling. Phenol peels, in particular, can result in skin lightening or darkening, which may be permanent in some cases.

SAFEGUARDING SENSITIVE SKIN TYPES

When getting chemical peels, sensitive skin needs to be treated with extra caution. First, a dermatologist should be consulted to determine the appropriate strength of the peel and to assess skin sensitivity. Superficial peels with gentle AHAs are generally a safer option for sensitive skin because they exfoliate the skin slightly without causing significant irritation.

Before a full peel, patch testing is advised to assess skin reactivity and verify compatibility with the peel solution; your dermatologist will closely monitor your skin throughout the procedure and alter the peel's intensity as needed.

Sensitive skin care after peeling includes moisturizing and washing gently, steering clear of harsh products and prolonged sun exposure, and using calming components like hyaluronic acid or aloe vera to relax the skin and encourage healing without aggravating sensitivity.

People with sensitive skin can safely benefit from chemical peels, attaining smoother, more radiant skin with a lower chance of negative reactions, by taking these measures and following these suggestions.

CHAPTER FOUR

BEFORE YOU BEGIN

MEETING WITH AN ESTHETICIAN OR DERMATOLOGIST

To ensure your safety and get the desired results from the peel, it is imperative that you first schedule a consultation with a qualified dermatologist or esthetician. During this consultation, the skin care professional will assess your skin type, talk about your skincare concerns, and go over your medical history to determine if you are a good candidate for a chemical peel. They will also go over the various types of peels that are available, from superficial to deep peels, and recommend the best one for your skin condition.

The dermatologist or esthetician will also answer any questions you may have and dispel any doubts you may have about the peel procedure. In addition, the consultation will set the stage for a safe and effective peel experience that is customized to your skin's unique needs and concerns. They will go over the potential benefits and risks associated with chemical peels, including potential side effects like redness, peeling, and temporary sensitivity. They will also provide detailed instructions on how to prepare for the peel, including any skincare products you should avoid in the days leading up to the treatment.

PRE-PEEL SKINCARE REGIMEN

Preparing your skin adequately before a chemical peel can significantly enhance the results and minimize the risk of complications. A pre-peel skincare regimen typically starts about two weeks before the scheduled treatment. The goal during this period is to optimize your skin's health and resilience, ensuring it is in the best possible condition to undergo the peel. Your dermatologist or esthetician may recommend gentle cleansers and moisturizers that are suitable for your skin type to maintain hydration and balance.

Additionally, they may advise you to discontinue the use of certain skincare products that could increase skin sensitivity, such as retinoids or exfoliating acids. Sunscreen becomes even more crucial during this time to protect your skin from UV damage, which can exacerbate post-peel complications like hyperpigmentation. Some professionals might also suggest incorporating calming ingredients like aloe vera or hyaluronic acid to soothe and hydrate the skin, preparing it for the exfoliation process ahead.

By diligently following this pre-peel skincare regimen, you not only help your skin tolerate the chemical peel better but also lay the foundation for more predictable and satisfactory results. This proactive approach ensures that your skin is as healthy and resilient as possible, minimizing the risk of adverse reactions and maximizing the benefits of the peel treatment.

SENSITIVITY TESTING AND PATCH TESTING

Before undergoing a chemical peel, it's essential to conduct patch testing and sensitivity checks to assess how your skin will react to the peel solution. This step helps identify any potential allergic reactions or extreme sensitivities that could complicate the peel procedure. Patch testing involves applying a small amount of the peel solution to a discreet area of your skin, such as behind your ear or on your forearm, and observing the skin's response over the next 24 to 48 hours.

You should keep a close eye on the patched area during this time for any unusual reactions, such as redness, swelling, itching, or other symptoms. If you do experience any discomfort or unfavorable reactions, you should notify your dermatologist or esthetician right away so they can modify the peel formulation or suggest other treatments that are more appropriate for your skin type.

Preparing for the transformative effects of a chemical peel by prioritizing patch testing and sensitivity checks helps ensure that your skin is in a stable condition for the peel and minimizes the risk of complications during and after the treatment.

Sensitivity checks also entail evaluating your skin's overall sensitivity by assessing factors such as recent sun exposure, existing skin conditions like eczema or rosacea, and any medications you may be taking.

MODIFICATIONS TO LIFESTYLE BOTH BEFORE AND AFTER PEELS

To maximize outcomes and encourage skin healing, there are specific lifestyle modifications that must be made before and following a chemical peel. First and foremost, you must minimize sun exposure and wear a broad-spectrum sunscreen every day to protect your skin from UV rays and lower your chances of developing hyperpigmentation or sunburn after the peel.

A balanced diet and adequate hydration support overall skin health and resilience; the former helps your skin recover more quickly after the peel and improves the efficacy of skincare products used during the healing process. In addition, you may need to stop using certain skincare products or treatments in the days preceding the peel, such as waxing or using abrasive exfoliants.

Following the peel, you should carefully adhere to the post-care instructions that your dermatologist or esthetician provides.

These instructions usually include moisturizing, cleansing gently, and applying skincare products that are recommended to promote healing and reduce inflammation. You may have mild discomfort, redness, or peeling after the peel, but these are normal side effects that usually go away in a few days to a week.

Following a chemical peel, sustaining the effects, and ensuring long-term skin health and renewal requires consistency in skincare and sun protection practices. By implementing these lifestyle choices, you create an ideal environment for your skin to recuperate and reap the full advantages of the peel.

SETTING OBJECTIVES AND CONTROLLING EXPECTATIONS

Chemical peels can address a variety of skin concerns, including acne scars, uneven skin tone, fine lines, and sun damage, but the extent of improvement may vary from person to person. Be honest about your skincare goals and concerns with your dermatologist or esthetician during your consultation. Setting realistic expectations and clearly defining your goals for the procedure is crucial before undergoing one.

They will evaluate the state of your skin and give you an honest assessment of what the peel can accomplish given your unique situation. It's critical to realize that chemical peels are not a one-size-fits-all treatment and may need several treatments to produce the desired outcomes, particularly for more complicated skin conditions.

In addition, it's important to know how long recovery times and possible downtime vary depending on the type of peel; deeper peels can cause more significant peeling and longer recovery periods. Your skincare professional will also provide you with information about what to expect both during and after the peel, including any temporary side effects and how to effectively manage them.

You can approach the chemical peel treatment with confidence and dedication to achieving healthier, more radiant skin by setting realistic goals and being aware of the process. Good communication with your dermatologist or esthetician guarantees that the treatment plan is customized to your unique needs and expectations, resulting in a positive and satisfying experience with long-lasting skincare benefits.

CHAPTER FIVE
CHEMICAL PEEL PROCEDURE
STEP-BY-STEP BREAKDOWN OF THE PROCEDURE

During a chemical peel, there are a few steps that must be followed to guarantee safety and efficacy. First, the skin needs to be thoroughly cleaned to eliminate any oils or impurities that might interfere with the peel's action. Next, the chemical solution that is customized for your skin type and treatment objectives is carefully applied. This application is usually done with a cotton applicator or gentle strokes to ensure even coverage while avoiding sensitive areas like the lips and eyes. Finally, the peel solution is left on for a specified amount of time following the application, based on the strength of the peel and your skin's reaction.

Knowing these procedural steps enables novices to participate confidently in the chemical peel process, guaranteeing the best results and skin rejuvenation.

After the exposure time, the peel solution is neutralized with a neutralizing agent or cool water to stop its activity and prevent over-exfoliation. Post-peel care then entails applying soothing creams or serums to hydrate and protect the skin, along with sunscreen to shield against UV damage.

WHAT TO ANTICIPATE FROM THE PEELING SESSION

You can expect a range of sensations and reactions during a chemical peel session as the peel solution interacts with your skin. If the peel is strong, you may experience temporary redness or flaking immediately after treatment, which is a normal part of the skin's renewal process. Initially, a mild tingling or warming sensation is common upon application, indicating the peel's activation. This sensation typically subsides as the peel progresses.

Additionally, some peels can hurt for a short while, especially in sensitive areas. However, most clinics provide comfort measures like cooling fans or numbing creams to help ease any discomfort during the procedure. You should discuss any discomfort you experience with your technician so they can make any necessary adjustments to the procedure. With this knowledge of expected sensations, beginners can go into their first peel session feeling confident and realistic about their skin's reaction.

PAIN CONTROL AND COMFORT MEASURES

Comfort during a chemical peel requires taking proactive steps to reduce any potential discomfort. A lot of clinics offer options like cooling packs or numbing creams before the peel application, which can help minimize pain and sensitivity. It's also important to keep lines of communication open with your technician so that adjustments in technique or solution strength can be made to improve comfort without sacrificing the effectiveness of the peel.

Following a peel, soothing masks or hydrating serums are frequently applied to calm the skin and enhance comfort.

These comfort measures not only improve the overall experience but also promote a positive outcome by supporting the skin's healing process and minimizing post-treatment redness or irritation. Additionally, implementing relaxation techniques during the procedure, such as deep breathing or listening to calming music, can further alleviate any anxiety or discomfort.

OBSERVING THE PEEL'S EFFECTS ON THE SKIN

Throughout the application process, your technician will monitor your skin's reaction to the peel solution, noting any immediate reactions like redness or mild irritation. They will also assess the depth of the peel's penetration and adjust accordingly to achieve desired results while protecting skin health. Skin reaction monitoring is critical to ensuring safety and efficacy during a chemical peel session.

In addition, post-peel monitoring entails assessing how your skin responds in the hours and days that follow treatment. Anticipated reactions could include transient redness, mild flaking, or elevated sensitivity, all of which are signs of the exfoliation process of the peel. By closely observing these reactions, technicians can offer customized post-care recommendations, like light cleansing and moisturizing regimens, to maximize recovery and improve skin rejuvenation.

GUIDELINES FOR TECHNICIANS OR SELF-APPLICATION

For professional treatments, technicians are trained to assess skin type and condition, choose the appropriate peel solution, and apply it safely and effectively. They follow strict protocols to ensure optimal results and minimize risks, such as allergic reactions or excessive irritation. Trained technicians can apply chemical peels in clinical settings or at home with appropriate guidance.

If self-application is something you're thinking about doing at home, though, make sure you carefully follow the manufacturer's instructions, which should include a patch test to determine skin tolerance before full application. Beginners should start with milder peel formulations and work their way up to a more potent formulation as they gain experience and understand how their skin responds to it. Applying the product according to the recommended dosage and following up with care instructions is crucial to getting results that are safe and effective, whether done by a technician or at home.

These thorough explanations provide novices a thorough grasp of what to anticipate and how to successfully navigate the chemical peel procedure, guaranteeing safety and the best possible results for skin renewal.

CHAPTER SIX

RECUPERATION AND AFTERCARE

QUICK POST-PEEL SKINCARE PROTOCOL

Immediately following a chemical peel, your skincare routine should be focused on hydrating and soothing the skin. Start by cleaning your face with a mild, non-abrasive cleanser to remove any debris or leftover peel solution. Avoid harsh scrubbing or exfoliation during this time to prevent irritation. Your skin will need special care to maximize healing and results following a chemical peel.

After peeling, apply a calming moisturizer rich in hydrating ingredients like ceramides or hyaluronic acid. These ingredients help to seal in moisture and provide a protective layer on the skin. Steer clear of products with strong chemicals or fragrances because your skin may be more sensitive after peeling.

Finally, to help protect your recently exposed skin from harmful UV rays and prevent further damage, don't forget to apply a broad-spectrum sunscreen with SPF 30 or higher, even when you're indoors. Adherence to these steps will help promote healing and effectively maintain the results of your chemical peel.

HANDLING PAIN AND REDNESS

It's normal to feel a little uncomfortable and a little red after a chemical peel, especially in the hours just after the treatment.

If you want to effectively manage these side effects, try applying a cool compress to your face to help relieve any burning sensations and minimize inflammation.

Avoid scratching or picking at your skin to prevent further irritation and possible infection. You can also take over-the-counter pain medicines like ibuprofen to help with discomfort, but always check with your healthcare professional before taking any medication after peeling.

Try putting on a light, moisturizing mask or using a moisturizer made especially for sensitive skin if your skin feels tight or dry. Look for products that have calming components like chamomile or aloe vera to relax the skin and reduce redness.

LONG-TERM SKINCARE THINGS TO THINK ABOUT

After the first peel recovery period, a long-term skincare regimen is essential to keeping skin healthy and looking refreshed. Use moderate cleansers and moisturizers suited to your skin type to avoid irritation and stay hydrated.

Incorporate exfoliation into your routine; however, to prevent overstripping your skin, use light chemical or enzyme-based exfoliants, which encourage cell turnover and maintain the appearance of luminous skin.

Consistency is crucial in skincare; to get the most out of your chemical peel, create a routine that you can stick to. Regular usage of serums containing antioxidants, such as vitamin C, can also assist in protecting your skin from environmental damage and sustain collagen synthesis.

PREVENTING SUN EXPOSURE AND USING SPF

Your skin is more vulnerable to UV radiation after a chemical peel, so you should try to limit your time spent in the sun, especially between the hours of 10 AM and 4 PM. When you are outside, wear protective gear like wide-brimmed hats and sunglasses, and look for shade whenever you can.

Even on overcast days or when inside near windows, use a broad-spectrum sunscreen with SPF 30 or higher every day. To maintain continuous protection, reapply sunscreen every two hours or right away after swimming or perspiring.

To prevent clogging pores or irritating sensitive skin, look for sunscreens that are designated as non-comedogenic. Proactive sun protection helps prolong the effects of chemical peels by preventing hyperpigmentation, premature aging, and other sun-induced skin damage.

INDICATIONS OF PROBLEMS AND WHEN TO GET ASSISTANCE

Chemical peels are generally safe, but it's important to be aware of any side effects. You should get in touch with your healthcare practitioner right away if you feel severe or persistent redness, swelling, or irritation that does not go away.

In the same way, if you notice any unusual changes in your skin's texture or color, or if your skin develops blisters or scabs, consult a healthcare professional for evaluation and appropriate management. Indicators of infection include increased pain, warmth, or pus-like discharge from treated areas.

Always adhere to your provider's post-peel care instructions and get in touch if you have any questions or concerns regarding your skin are healing process.

CHAPTER SEVEN

TYPICAL FEARS REGARDING CHEMICAL PEELS

SAFETY ISSUES AND MYTHS DISPELLED

Safety is the most important consideration when it comes to chemical peels. There are a few common misconceptions and concerns that often discourage novices from attempting these procedures. Firstly, there is a common misconception that chemical peels are only for severe skin issues. While they can address serious concerns like acne scars or hyperpigmentation, there are milder peels suitable for beginners seeking a fresher complexion. Modern chemical peels are designed to be safe and effective when performed by a trained professional.

Ignore these myths and learn the safety protocols so that beginners can approach chemical peels with confidence and achieve smoother, rejuvenated skin. To ensure safety during a chemical peel, choose a qualified skincare professional or dermatologist.

They will assess your skin type and recommend the appropriate peel strength. Unlike other treatments, chemical peels are customized to your skin's needs, minimizing risks like excessive redness or irritation. Consistently following pre- and post-peel care instructions is also important to maximize safety and achieve the desired results.

HANDLING SENSATIONS AFTER PEELING

Understanding and coping with these sensations is essential for a positive experience following a chemical peel. Immediately following the peel, you might feel a slight tingling or warmth as the solution penetrates the skin; this sensation will soon go away, and it's normal for your skin to appear slightly flushed. Your skincare professional can recommend cooling and hydrating masks to help ease any discomfort.

It's common to experience mild flaking or peeling, especially with deeper peels. Gentle exfoliation using recommended products can assist in removing dead skin cells gently. By understanding and managing these post-peel sensations, beginners can support their skin's healing process and achieve optimal results from the treatment. In the days following a peel, your skin may feel tighter than usual as it begins to shed dead cells. This process is essential for revealing fresher skin underneath.

HANDLING TRANSIENT SKIN CHANGES

Beginners should expect temporary changes to their skin as part of the chemical peel process. Depending on the strength of the peel, your skin may appear red or blotchy immediately after the procedure; this redness usually goes away in a few hours to a day. For deeper peels, you may notice visible peeling over several days as the skin sheds its outer layers; this is normal and shows that the peel was effective in promoting skin renewal.

After a peel, some novices may experience more sensitivity to sunlight. To protect the newly exposed skin layers, it's important to apply sunscreen religiously and avoid prolonged sun exposure. Hydration is crucial during this time to maintain skin moisture and support the healing process. Using gentle, non-irritating skincare products that your skincare professional recommends will help minimize discomfort and maximize the benefits of the peel. By being aware of these temporary changes and planning appropriately, novices can successfully navigate the post-peel phase and attain smoother, healthier skin.

MANAGING SURPRISING REACTIONS

Mild reactions can include increased redness, itching, or a burning sensation during or immediately after the peel; these symptoms usually go away quickly with proper post-peel care, such as applying soothing creams or cold compresses as recommended. Unexpected reactions to chemical peels are rare, but they can happen, especially for beginners with sensitive skin.

More severe reactions, such as blistering or extended redness, are rare but can happen.

If you have any of these symptoms, it's important to get in touch with your skincare specialist right away so they can evaluate the situation and suggest treatments that will help reduce discomfort and encourage healing. Beginners can reduce risks and guarantee a safe experience with chemical peels that are customized to their skin's needs by being alert and responsive to unexpected reactions.

GETTING READY FOR SEVERAL PEEL SESSIONS

When starting a chemical peel regimen for the first time, it's important to plan on needing multiple sessions to achieve the desired results. The frequency and intensity of peels vary depending on the goals and conditions of each client.

It may be suggested to start with a series of lighter peels spaced several weeks apart to give your skin time to adjust. This will reduce the chance of negative reactions and optimize the benefits of each treatment.

Following your skin care professional's pre-peel instructions is crucial before each session. Usually, this entails avoiding sun exposure, stopping certain skincare products, and getting your skin ready for the treatment. Aftercare is just as important to support skin healing and extend the results. Regular skin care routines, such as moisturizing and protecting your skin from the sun, will help maintain the improvements made with each peel session.

A skincare professional will modify the peel strength or formulation as you go through multiple peel sessions to address changing skin needs and goals; sharing any concerns or changes in your skin's response is essential to maximizing treatment results. With careful planning and expert guidance, novices can successfully navigate multiple peel sessions, obtaining progressive and noticeable improvements in skin texture and appearance.

CHAPTER EIGHT

SELECTING AN EXPERT OR DO IT YOURSELF METHOD

BENEFITS AND DRAWBACKS OF EXPERT TREATMENTS

In addition to using higher concentrations of acids that can penetrate deeper layers of the skin to target specific concerns like acne scars, fine lines, and hyperpigmentation more effectively, professional chemical peels offer several advantages for those seeking advanced skincare treatments. One of the main benefits is the expertise provided by trained professionals who assess your skin type and tailor the peel accordingly. Professionals also ensure safety during the procedure, minimizing the risk of adverse reactions through proper application and post-peel care.

Professional treatments do have some disadvantages, though. Because they require specialized training and equipment, they are usually more expensive than do-it-yourself options. Making appointments can be time-consuming, especially if multiple sessions are required to achieve desired results. Some people may also experience discomfort during or after the peel, such as temporary sensitivity to sunlight, redness, or swelling. Despite these potential drawbacks, many people prefer professional treatments because they are efficient and come with the assurance of expert care.

SELF-MADE PEEL KITS: THEIR PERFORMANCE

Convenience and affordability are the main draws for DIY chemical peel kits. These kits typically contain lactic or glycolic acid in lower concentrations, which are milder acids meant for at-home use without professional supervision. Applying these kits is relatively simple if you follow the instructions, and they can gradually improve the texture and tone of your skin. DIY kits are also a good option for people with busy schedules who would rather treat their skin in the comfort of their own homes.

A patch test should be performed before full application to determine skin tolerance and adjust usage accordingly. DIY peel kits can be very effective, but their effectiveness varies depending on the concentration of acids and individual skin sensitivity. Although they can offer mild exfoliation and superficial improvement, they may not be as effective at addressing deep-seated skin issues as professional treatments.

SAFETY MEASURES FOR PEELS AT HOME

When using chemical peels at home, safety must always come first. Before using any product, make sure you read and comprehend all of the instructions. Do a patch test on a small area of skin to check for allergies or adverse reactions. Always apply the peel according to the recommended time. Do not leave the peel on longer than necessary to avoid burns or irritation.

When applying, it's best to wear safety goggles and gloves to protect the hands and eyes from potentially harmful acids. You should also make sure the room has enough ventilation to release any fumes from the chemical solution. After peeling, use a mild cleanser and moisturizer meant for post-peel care to help heal the skin and speed up the healing process. If you experience any extreme reactions—like severe burning or blistering—you should go to the doctor right away.

SPEAKING WITH SKINCARE PROFESSIONALS

It is highly recommended that you speak with a skincare expert before beginning a chemical peel regimen, especially if you are new to the process. Skincare experts can evaluate your skin type, current conditions, and specific concerns to recommend the best type of peel. They can also offer helpful advice on how to prepare your skin in advance as well as what to expect during and after the treatment.

In addition to offering customized peel treatments based on your skin's needs, experts can also offer advice on supplementary skincare products and routines to maintain skin health in between treatments and maximize results without needless risks. Consultations also provide an opportunity to ask questions about potential side effects, downtime, and long-term skincare goals, enabling you to make well-informed decisions about your skincare regimen.

COST COMPARISONS AND BUDGETARY CONSIDERATIONS

Budget is a crucial consideration when deciding between professional and do-it-yourself chemical peels. Professional peels can vary in price depending on the type of peel, the location of the clinic, and the practitioner's level of experience. The cost may also increase if multiple sessions are needed to achieve the desired results.

DIY peel kits are typically less expensive upfront because they do not require professional services or clinic visits; however, continuous peel kit purchases can add up over time, particularly if repeat treatments are required. It is important to compare the long-term costs of both options, taking into account not only the financial implications but also the convenience and expected results. Selecting the best course of action requires striking a balance between budgetary constraints and desired skincare outcomes.

CHAPTER NINE

ADVANCED ADVICE FOR BETTER OUTCOMES

When experimenting with chemical peels for skincare, it's important to think about how these procedures can work in concert with other skincare regimens. For example, combining peels with complementary procedures like face masks or serums can improve overall skin rejuvenation. Applying a hydrating mask after a peel can help calm the skin and restore moisture that was lost during the exfoliation process. Alternatively, applying a vitamin C serum before a peel can prepare the skin by increasing the production of collagen, which will maximize the effectiveness of the peel.

In addition, combining peels with daily skincare practices like cleansing and moisturizing promotes long-term skin health and resilience.

This method not only prepares the skin for peels but also keeps it intact in between treatments. By carefully planning peels into an all-encompassing skincare regimen, people can attain more significant and durable outcomes, effectively addressing a range of skin concerns.

ENHANCING PEEL PERFORMANCE WITH COMPLEMENTARY ITEMS

To get the most out of chemical peels, you must pair them with appropriate skincare products. For example, cleaning the skin with a mild exfoliant before the peel can help the solution go deeper into the skin, and using a calming moisturizer afterward can help the skin regain its moisture and reduce irritation, which will speed up healing and improve overall outcomes.

By choosing the right products that work synergistically with peels, people can make sure that their skin receives optimal nourishment and protection throughout the treatment process.

Furthermore, using products enriched with antioxidants like vitamin E or green tea extract can protect the skin from free radicals and oxidative stress, which can compromise the benefits of chemical peels. These antioxidants also support skin healing and collagen synthesis, crucial for maintaining skin health after peeling sessions.

CUSTOMIZING PEELS TO ADDRESS PARTICULAR SKIN ISSUES

A customized approach based on individual skin types and conditions is necessary when adapting chemical peels to address particular skin concerns. For instance, salicylic acid peels can be beneficial for acne-prone skin because they effectively unclog pores and reduce acne lesions; on the other hand, glycolic acid peels can promote cellular turnover and fade pigmentation in sun-damaged skin.

In addition, different levels of skin sensitivity and treatment objectives can be accommodated by varying the intensity and frequency of peels.

It is important to consult a skin care professional to find the best type and concentration of peel for a given concern. By personalizing peel treatments, people can attain specific outcomes like improved tone, smoother texture, and overall more radiant skin that are catered to their skincare needs.

REGULARITY OF PEEL PROCEDURES

The optimal frequency of chemical peel treatments depends on the patient's skin type and desired level of resurfacing. In general, novices should begin with less intense peels spaced a few weeks apart to give their skin time to adjust and heal completely in between treatments.

As tolerance and skin response improves, progressively increasing the frequency or intensity of peels can result in more noticeable and durable results.

Peel intervals should be followed as prescribed by a professional to avoid over-exfoliation and reduce the risk of adverse reactions like redness or irritation. Using sunscreen and moisturizing in between treatments will help keep skin healthy and extend the benefits of chemical peels. Patients can gradually improve their skin's texture, tone, and appearance by following a treatment plan that is consistent with their skincare objectives.

SUSTAINING SKIN HEALTH IN BETWEEN APPOINTMENTS

Achieving long-lasting results and reducing risks requires maintaining optimal skin health in between chemical peel sessions. Using non-irritating skincare products customized for each type of skin type ensures continuous hydration and nourishment, promoting overall resilience to peel treatments. Developing a daily skincare routine that includes sun protection, cleansing, and moisturizing helps to preserve skin integrity.

Furthermore, hydrating masks or serums added to weekly skincare rituals can further improve skin hydration and barrier function, supporting recovery and maintaining a healthy complexion in between peel sessions. As UV damage can undo the benefits of chemical peels and exacerbate skin sensitivity, protecting the skin from UV damage is crucial.

People can maximize the results of chemical peel treatments by making consistent skincare practices a priority and following the post-peel instructions that skincare professionals provide. By taking preventative measures, people can maintain the health of their skin while also increasing the efficacy and durability of the results, which will eventually leave their complexion looking refreshed and smooth.

CHAPTER TEN

COMMON QUESTIONS AND EXTENSIVE ANSWERS

TAKING CARE OF SAFETY AND SIDE EFFECTS ISSUES

When it comes to chemical peels, safety is the most important factor, especially for first-timers. It is important to see a dermatologist to determine your skin type and any underlying conditions that may affect the outcome of the peel. Common side effects include temporary redness, peeling, and mild irritation, which usually go away in a few days. Serious side effects, such as infection or scarring, are rare but possible, which emphasizes the need for professional application and aftercare.

Those who follow these precautions and choose a reputable provider can safely enjoy the benefits of chemical peels. Proper preparation entails stopping the use of certain skincare products or medications that could heighten sensitivity to the peel.

During the procedure, a trained practitioner applies the peel solution evenly to the skin, which may cause a tingling or mild burning sensation. Post-peel care involves gentle cleansing and moisturizing to promote healing and protect the newly revealed skin.

SELECTING THE APPROPRIATE PEEL STRENGTH

A beginner should begin with mild peels, such as superficial or light peels, which gently exfoliate the skin's outer layer without causing significant downtime. These peels are suitable for addressing minor texture irregularities, fine lines, and mild discoloration. The appropriate strength of the peel depends on individual skin concerns and desired outcomes.

Deep peels are only recommended for experienced users and dermatologist-administered treatments due to their intense exfoliating properties and potential for significant downtime. Medium peels, on the other hand, penetrate deeper into the skin and are effective for treating moderate discoloration, wrinkles, and acne scars. However, they may require a longer recovery period and can cause more noticeable peeling and redness.

Gradually increasing peel strength allows beginners to acclimate their skin and achieve optimal outcomes with each session. Speaking with a skincare professional is essential to determine the most suitable peel strength based on skin type, sensitivity, and specific concerns. They can also recommend a personalized treatment plan that maximizes results while minimizing potential risks and discomfort.

DRUG PEELS AND PREGNANCY

Pregnancy-related risks include the possibility of harm to the fetus as well as the absorption of certain chemicals from chemical peels, like glycolic acid and salicylic acid, into the bloodstream; however, there is a lack of conclusive research on the safety of these chemicals during pregnancy.

Pregnancy is a time when most healthcare providers advise against deep or medium chemical peels; instead, they suggest gentler alternatives like topical skincare products with safe concentrations of exfoliating agents, which can help maintain skin texture and clarity without the risks of professional chemical peels.

Making educated decisions about skincare treatments during pregnancy requires prioritizing prenatal care and speaking with a healthcare provider. If a peel is considered medically necessary during pregnancy, it should only be done by a qualified healthcare professional who can minimize exposure to potentially harmful ingredients and ensure adequate safety measures.

EFFECTS ON SKIN HEALTH OVER TIME

Regular application of mild to moderate peels can stimulate collagen production, reducing the appearance of fine lines and improving skin elasticity over time.

Although chemical peels provide immediate benefits, such as improved skin texture and tone, understanding their long-term effects is essential for maintaining healthy skin.

But too frequent or too aggressive peels can damage the skin's natural protective layer, causing more irritation, dryness, and redness. It's crucial to space out peel treatments by professional guidelines so that the skin has enough time to heal in between treatments.

In addition, proper post-peel care—using sunscreen and moisturizing the skin—helps preserve the results of chemical peels over time and helps prevent hyperpigmentation and acne scarring, which can lead to a more even complexion and smoother skin texture.

HOW TO INCLUDE PEELS IN YOUR DAILY SKINCARE REGIMEN

A consultation with a skincare professional is the first step in incorporating chemical peels into a skincare routine; during this consultation, skin health will be assessed and the most suitable type and frequency of peels will be determined.

On the day of the peel, carefully clean the skin to eliminate oil and grime to ensure that the peel solution adheres uniformly. Before arranging a peel, prepare the skin by stopping the use of retinoids and exfoliating agents to minimize any irritation and sensitivity.

After the peel, replenish moisture and soothe any redness or irritation caused by the peel by using hydrating serums and soothing masks; these steps may include light cleansing, moisturizing, and daily use of a broad-spectrum sunscreen. These post-procedure instructions will be given to you by your skincare professional.

CHAPTER ELEVEN
TRENDS IN CHEMICAL PEELS GOING FORWARD
NOVELTIES IN PEEL COMBINATIONS

The skincare industry has seen a revolution in recent years with the introduction of safer and more effective peel formulations that provide solutions for skin rejuvenation. The focus of these innovations has been on improving efficacy while minimizing side effects, with a particular focus on novices in the field of chemical peels. The gentler acids, like lactic acid or mandelic acid, are well-suited for sensitive skin types and less likely to cause post-peel complications like redness or irritation. Additionally, buffered solutions that maintain a stable pH throughout the application ensure consistent results without jeopardizing the integrity of the skin barrier.

Furthermore, targeted peel formulations have been developed to address particular skincare issues like hyperpigmentation, acne scars, and fine lines.

This customization enables practitioners to customize treatments based on patient needs, which maximizes results for first-time chemical peel patients. Furthermore, advancements in peel delivery systems, like ingredients that are encapsulated and penetrate deeper layers of the skin, improve treatment outcomes while reducing application discomfort.

Those who are new to the world of chemical peels will find that knowing about these advancements helps them make educated decisions and feel more confident about the safety and efficacy of the treatment. Adding these innovations to their skincare regimens improves the overall experience and results in healthier, more radiant skin.

NEW DEVELOPMENTS IN SKINCARE TECHNOLOGY

The use of cutting-edge technologies in skin rejuvenation has broadened the range of treatment options available to novices contemplating chemical peels. Non-invasive options such as laser-assisted peels and ultrasound devices offer a substitute for traditional chemical peel techniques, giving precise control over treatment depth and addressing particular skin concerns. These innovations reduce recovery time and discomfort, opening up skin rejuvenation to a wider range of people looking for gentle yet effective solutions.

Moreover, light-based therapies like LED and IPL (Intense Pulsed Light) treatments augment chemical peels by augmenting collagen production and refining overall skin texture. These technologies not only expedite healing but also extend the outcomes of chemical peel treatments, bolstering skin health for novices starting their skincare journey. Moreover, developments in digital imaging and skin analysis tools empower professionals to precisely diagnose skin conditions, enabling customized treatment regimens and tracking advancements over time.

Beginning with these new technologies, beginners can discover cutting-edge skincare methods that put safety, effectiveness, and patient satisfaction first. Acknowledging these developments guarantees a thorough approach to skin rejuvenation, enabling people to attain long-lasting improvements in their skin tone, texture, and overall appearance.

ECO-FRIENDLY METHODS IN PEEL MANUFACTURING

Sustainable peel formulations prioritize biodegradable ingredients and cruelty-free testing methods, aligning with consumer preferences for ethically sourced skincare products. Manufacturers are increasingly adopting eco-friendly ingredients and packaging materials, minimizing carbon footprints and reducing waste throughout the production process. Sustainable peel manufacturing practices have become increasingly important in shaping the future of the skincare industry in response to growing environmental awareness.

In addition, new developments in manufacturing technologies emphasize the use of renewable resources and energy-efficient processes, encouraging ethical behavior without sacrificing the quality of the product. These initiatives meet consumer demand for chemical peels while also supporting conservation efforts and reducing environmental impact. Sustainable packaging options, like recyclable containers and simple designs, also help to create a circular economy in the beauty industry.

Aware of these sustainable practices encourages environmentally conscious consumer choices and fosters environmental stewardship, even for novices exploring chemical peels. Adopting sustainable skincare options not only supports healthier skin but also makes a global contribution to efforts to preserve natural resources for future generations.

TEACHING MATERIALS FOR CONTINUOUS EDUCATION

To ensure safe and successful treatment outcomes, beginners navigating the world of chemical peels need to have access to comprehensive educational resources. These resources offer essential knowledge and practical insights into treatment protocols and skincare practices through courses, workshops, and webinars led by industry experts. Topics covered include peel formulations and application techniques, post-treatment care, and patient management.

Additionally, peer-to-peer learning and mentorship opportunities are made possible by online forums and professional networks, which enable novices to share experiences, ask questions, and remain informed about the most recent developments in skincare and dermatology.

Interactive educational resources, like case studies and virtual simulations, improve learning retention and skill development and prepare practitioners for a variety of clinical scenarios and patient interactions.

In the case of novices in chemical peels, making use of these educational resources encourages ongoing education and career development, boosting self-assurance in providing superior skincare services.

Living lifelong learning embraces clinical proficiency and builds patient confidence and satisfaction, laying the groundwork for a prosperous skincare and dermatology career.

INTERNATIONAL VIEWS OF SKINCARE TRENDS

Gaining an understanding of the various viewpoints on skincare trends around the world can help novices learn about cultural preferences, local skincare practices, and new market opportunities about chemical peels. As different regions prioritize different skincare concerns, different formulations and treatment approaches for different skin types and environmental conditions are adopted. For example, Asian markets drive innovation in peel formulations that are enhanced with antioxidants and botanical extracts, while also emphasizing brightening and anti-aging benefits.

Global skincare trends also draw attention to the increasing need for sustainable skincare solutions and inclusive beauty standards, which are driving the development of eco-friendly and ethical practices in the industry. Different market dynamics, such as consumer preferences and regulatory frameworks, affect product formulation strategies and marketing approaches for chemical peels across continents. By comprehending these global viewpoints, novices can modify their business strategies and skincare practices to become competitive and relevant in the global market.

Furthermore, the skincare industry benefits from cross-cultural collaborations and knowledge exchange initiatives that foster innovation and diversity in peel manufacturing and treatment modalities. By adopting global perspectives, novices can acquire a comprehensive understanding of consumer behaviors and skincare trends, which in turn promotes strategic growth and well-informed decision-making in the highly competitive chemical peel market.

www.ingramcontent.com/pod-product-compliance
Lightning Source LLC
Chambersburg PA
CBHW061258250726

48653CB00002B/678